Lose Weight FAST

Secrets to Losing Weight & Keeping It Off

By

Joshua Randolph

TABLE OF CONTENTS

INTRODUCTION

How many of us can honestly say that we have had our share of diet rollercoasters? You know those types of diets where you do good for a minute and then suddenly you fall right back off. It's like you go through the up and down stage in the same manner a rollercoaster goes through it's up and down motions.

While the rollercoaster is an amusement, it's not so much that way on the weight loss side. The multiple ups and downs can leave a person feeling depleted and can cause them to give up totally.

That's the reason I decided to write this book. I too was in that place of frustration. I was tired of the rollercoasters I was experiencing; while trying my best to live healthy and fit. Every time I took one step forward it seemed like I got pushed four steps back.

That was until I came across this solution that has helped me lose 50lbs in just under 4 months while revolutionizing my entire life. I hope as you read this book you will have the same experience I have. It's time to not only lose weight, but to also lose it fast and keep it off for good!

Lose Weight FAST

& Keep It OFF

Chapter 1

The Wake-Up Call

There I was, walking through Walmart feeling down and very frustrated. Everything I was trying to do to lose weight and get back in shape wasn't working. I tried different meal prep plans, to different advice I would get from people in the gym. No matter what it was it seemed not to work for me. It left me very frustrated and down. I was tired of being in the position I was in and I needed help!

Not to mention I was battling Type 2 Diabetes as well. So not only was I trying to get back in shape, but I was also trying to get my sugar levels under control and hopefully off the medicines I was taking at the time. So many thoughts were going through my mind as I found myself walking down the aisles of Walmart.

I began to have the "why me" attitude. The attitude that says, "why me, why am I going through this?" "Why did this have to happen to me?" Why, why, why? As I pondered on those thoughts something strange clicked in my mind, I heard these words loud and clear "WHY NOT YOU?" It was as though God was telling me, why not you Josh? How do you know that I'm not using this situation to not only change your life but also the lives of many others?

I stood there shocked and amazed at the same time. I no longer felt down as I did when I first came to the store. I kind of felt encouraged and empowered. It was like a wake-up call or shall I say a call to action. I knew then that this was bigger than me, there was a bigger picture attached to this entire situation.

I began to hold my head up and say within myself, "okay Josh, it's time to man up and make this happen." I began to encourage myself right there in the store. My mind began to shift into more of a conqueror mindset rather than a defeated mindset. I began to see not only myself overcoming this weight loss problem, but many others as well.

I knew this was going to be a journey and not just a quick fix. I believe that's one of the major hiccups many people fall into. They look more to getting a quick fix than they do to doing the necessary things on a consistent basis that will produce a more longevity reward. The journey is what produces the character one will need in order to stay in the desired reward longer.

I walked down the aisle and began to ask God to show me what I needed to do and to give me direct instructions so I could begin to implement them into my life. After I prayed that simple prayer you won't believe what happened next. Let's just say God answered me quickly!

I began to walk to the part of the store where I would get my normal protein cookies and other protein products. After getting a few boxes of the cookies I began to walk to the register. Suddenly, a guy that I see at the gym all the time just so happen to walk pass me. Me being the kind person that I am I spoke to him. After shaking hands, I noticed he had a bunch of canned chicken products in his basket and some other health products.

In my curiosity I asked him why he had all those canned chicken products in his basket. Little did I know, God was about to change my entire life with his response. He went on to say, "Man bro., I changed my entire diet years ago and haven't looked back. I used to be 240lbs and I was fighting many health problems at the time. I had tried many things to get right and nothing worked for me. That's when I found out about intermediate fasting and it totally changed my entire life."

I was not only shocked by his response, but what was even more amazing to me was the fact that God placed this person in my life who was at a place physically I wanted to be. Also, he had been at a place I currently was but had overcome. You can imagine that I was all ears at this point. I wanted to know what his big secret was and how I could implement it and begin to see similar results.

I felt a level of comfort with him and began to share with him my situation and the physical struggles I was having. He sat there and listened intently to me and you could tell that he truly cared. After a few minutes of me sharing my frustrations with him he glanced down in my basket and began to smile. I was wondering what was funny, so I asked. He responded, "Bro. I see one of the problems already". He grabbed the two boxes of protein cookies, picked them up and smiled while he said, "These are your number one enemy."

I began to give him a confused look and I can tell he recognized it because he smiled and said, "I know they say "protein", but you have to realize that the amount of carbs you intake with one cookie is to much for what you are desiring to do." I asked him to explain and his response blew my mind. He said, "I too use to battle with Type 2 Diabetes, and I had to cut back on carbs tremendously. I found out that carbs were my number one enemy and I had to know how to fight it. That's when I found out about intermediate fasting. I began to cut my carb intake and I began to follow intermediate fasting which gave my body time to rest and recover. That is what totally changed my life."

I stood there in amazement. Not so much by what he had just spoken to me but more so by the way God had placed this person in the right spot at the right time. I was literally looking in the mirror at someone who had been through what I was going through. That alone made me appreciate God on a whole new level. I never really understood what my grandparents and parents meant by, "He may not be there when you want Him, but He will always be right on time", but after this experience I truly understood now.

He began to break down a game plan for me and told me that if I needed any assistance that he wouldn't mind helping me out. After hearing everything that he had shared with me I was extremely encouraged and ready to embark upon this lifechanging journey. Just in case you wondered, yes, I did put the protein cookies back lol.

Chapter 2
New Beginnings

Riding home that night was very uplifting. I had a plan in place, and I had the motivation needed to begin this journey. I can't lie though, there was a voice in the back of my head that was trying to tell me that this wouldn't work. I had to put that thought under me and not allow it to cause me to get discouraged. I knew deep down inside that something had to change, and I believed that this new-found information was going to be part of my change. I was determined to not allow anything, any thought, or any person stop me from getting what I desired.

Since this was going to be a new venture for me, I knew I had to also tighten things up spiritually and mentally. Many people lose the battle in their mind even before they get to the actual battle. A favorite quote of mine is, "As a man think, so is he." You will eventually become whatever you spend the most time thinking about. Negative thoughts will produce negative results just like positive thoughts will produce positive results.

I knew I couldn't allow anything negative or sabotaging into my mind and if it tried to creep in, I had to immediately cast it down. This caused me to come up with a spiritual plan as well. I not only wanted to deal with the physical side of my issue, but I also wanted to be able to deal with the whole me. I've learned through trial and error that to many times we focus on one area of our life and neglect other areas. This leaves us unbalanced and possibly sets us up for an even greater fall.

God had been dealing with me for a while to begin to get up early and pray, read my word, and meditate. Though I kept having these urges to do it something would always come up that would cause me to keep putting it off. Sometimes I ask myself, "what if this have been Gods way of trying to get my attention but I just wasn't listening." I knew for this new-found journey to work I had to also implement the getting up early portion as well.

So, there I was, pulling back into my driveway from the store with a solid plan. A bold level of determination rose up in me and I knew that it was going to work. Even though physically nothing had changed, mentally I had already begun to see myself in the place I desired to be. I finally saw the "New Me" in my mind.

One of my favorite scriptures comes to mind, Mark 11:24 says, "Therefore I say to you, whatever things you ask when you pray, believe that you receive them, and you will have them." Something amazing happens when you begin to believe you are already in the place you desire to be. When your mind begins to already see yourself there you begin to make better choices. You begin to choose to be around like-minded people, places, and things that will elevate you to higher levels of excellence. You no longer will accept a defeated mindset and you will no longer put up with mediocracy.

As I walked into the house my wife noticed that I had a look on my face. She asked why I was looking all happy and stuff. She jokingly asked if someone tried to flirt with me at the store lol. I smiled and said no and proceeded to share with her the encounter I had just experienced. My wife was so happy for me and said she will be there to help in any way possible.

I was ready to tackle my first day to a new me. That night I sat my workout clothes out and got everything ready for my new journey. I knew that I had to continue to work out, so I made sure to add that in my journey plans. I really didn't do much cardio up into this time, but I knew in order for this to work I had to do things that made me uncomfortable.

To many times people want to experience success while remaining in a comfort zone. I'm sorry to burst your bubble but that's called living in a fantasy. Anything worth having should always cause you to be willing and ready to become uncomfortable. It's in that place that you discover things about yourself that you didn't know existed. It's like tapping into the sleeping giant on the inside of you.

Trust me, I know new beginnings can be a little scary and even intimidating at times, but we must never be afraid to embrace these new beginnings. Sometimes just in you taking that first step you will realize that you were built for this.

Most of the successful people you see in the world today reached their level of success from an uncomfortable place. Either they were faced with some type of catastrophe like a death in the family or even the threat of foreclosure or eviction. Whatever the case may have been, it was in those moments of being uncomfortable that caused them to tap into a part of them that they didn't realize existed.

Whether you believe it our not, you also have a sleeping giant on the inside of you that's waiting to be tapped into. There is a creative genius inside of you cheering you on and waiting for you to tag him/her in so they can take your life to greatness. From this moment on never be afraid to embrace being uncomfortable for a season. The temporary pain will be worth the eternal reward if you choose not to quit.

Chapter 3

Plan in Motion

Beep, beep, beep! "Who in the world is that", as I thought to myself looking for my phone. As I grabbed my phone and saw that it was 3am in the morning I came to my senses and realized that it was the time I had set to get up and start my journey. I jumped up because I knew if I had hit the snooze button I wasn't going to get up. Funny thing is I didn't even feel sleepy and there was a burst of energy that I had never felt before.

After brushing my teeth, I grabbed my work-out clothes and headed down stairs. I was excited and nervous at the same time. This was something new for me, but I was determined to make this work. I knew that God had orchestrated my every step and I knew He was about to do something amazing in my body, mind, and spirit.

I made some tea and then went straight into prayer. This prayer time was different than any other prayer time that I've ever experienced. It was as though I was hearing God clearer than I have ever heard him. The experience was so awesome that I began to think within myself if this was the place God had been trying so long to get me to. I felt God speaking to my heart and mind and I felt Him encouraging me in a way that made me feel like superman.

After what seemed like hours in prayer, (even though it was only about 25 minutes) I got up and started reading my Bible. I would read a few scriptures and so many ideas were coming to me at once. I felt like a computer that was getting an upgrade on all its equipment. I began to write many of the ideas down and it was like they just kept coming. Before I knew it, I looked at the clock and it was almost 5am. I was like, WOW, that time flew past.

There's a saying that goes, "time flies by when you are having fun." I can now attest to that in a whole new spectrum. Our ideology doesn't have to always equate to "fun" as being parties, getting drunk, or just hanging out. Fun can and will happen as you tap into your potential and begin to do what you were called to do. I found myself having so much fun in this new journey that time just seemed like it flew passed.

Now that I had experienced the beginning stage of the mental and spiritual part of this new journey, it was time to experience the physical side. I had never been to the gym that early (5am) so this was something new for me and very uncomfortable. Not to mention I really wasn't a big fan of cardio. No matter how I felt about it I knew I had to attack this part of my life.

I once heard a person say, "What you refuse to conquer will eventually come back and conquer you". Wow! This is such a bold and true statement. Just because you ignore something doesn't mean that it will go away. That's like pulling the cover over your head hoping that the monster will go away. The problem with this is the fact that the so-called monster isn't the problem, THE FEAR OF THE MONSTER IS!

If you never identify what the real problem is, you will never be able to confront the thing that's trying to hold you back. Without the ability to "confront" you end up finding yourself just going through life without ever experiencing what it feels like to conquer. You were born to always conquer. That doesn't mean that you will never face tough challenges or even lose some battles, but you must know and believe that you were created to always conquer.

As I walked into the gym, I saw many other people coming in at 5am. That gave me encouragement and motivation. This was my first time coming to the gym at that time, but I was so ready to face this giant. I already had a game plan, 30 minutes on the stair master and 15 minutes in the sauna. I walked to that stair master machine with the mindset that this was going to be a piece of cake. Oh, how I was so wrong about that lol.

When I started off, I put the machine on level three and pressed start. For motivation I decided not to listen to music but to Dr. Bill Winston Ministries app. I figured that I could get some teaching and cardio at the same time. It started off very good but ten-minutes later I was sweating like never before and it felt like my chest was about to explode. It's funny to me now as I write this, but it wasn't funny at the time.

This taught me that in life some things may be easier than others, but eventually everything works together for our good. Let's take baking a cake for instance, many people love eating various types of cake. Me being a semi baker I know a thing or two about baking cakes (I say semi because I only know how to bake box cakes lol).

It takes different ingredients to be compounded into the cake in order for it to reach its highest level of the desired taste. Leave one ingredient out and it may not reach the level of excellence you desired it to reach. Try eating each ingredient separately and you may be in for a big surprise. Let me give you a hint, it won't taste like a cake lol. It takes ALL ingredients to come collectively together and work together to produce the tasteful cake you desired it to be.

The same thing applies to life. Everything we go through is truly working together for our good. Yes, EVERYTHING! The good and the bad, the ups and the downs. It may not feel like it at times, especially as we are in the midst of the storm, but we must realize that no matter what, it's still working out for our good!

Even though it felt like I was about to literally die I still refused to stop taking the next step. I was looking at the time every second, sweat dripping down my face and me constantly telling myself "don't stop, don't stop". Finally, it reached 30 minutes and I couldn't have been happier. I did it! I completed my first morning of fasted cardio and though I was extremely exhausted it felt good because I did it.

As I headed to the sauna, I turned some worship music on and began to meditate on positive things that I wanted to begin to experience in my life. I made up in my mind to make the most of this journey and to protect my peace with nothing but positive thoughts. The sauna felt very good after a 30-minute cardio work out. Though this may seem like a small accomplishment to some, to me it was a huge leap. I accomplished my first day with flying colors.

Later that night I went back to the gym for my normal work out. In order to achieve my goal, I knew I would have to work out twice a day. Therefore, I chose to do my cardio in the morning and my weight training at night. It was strenuous, but I knew this is what it was going to take. That night after my work out I ate a light meal and began to prepare for day two.

Chapter 4

Beware of SCUD'S

Anytime you make up in your mind that you are going to do something about the direction of your life BEWARE! Now before you get all fearful this isn't a tactic to try to scare you or deter you away from your goal. No, this is just a friendly insight to let you know that there is a true enemy out there and their job is to keep you from any progressive movement.

So, what is a SCUD? Satan Constantly Using Distractions. Distractions comes in many different shapes and sizes. They can come from watching too much TV or spending too much time on social media. They can also come from purposely surrounding yourself around mediocre and complacent people. No matter how they come or from whom they come you must believe THEY WILL COME!

First day was complete and I was ready to tackle the second day. As my alarm clock went off at 3am I jumped up and was excited about the time I was about to spend in prayer and meditation. Just like day one I got a lot out of the prayer and meditation time. As 5am began to approach I prepared for the gym.

Walking out of my house I was more prepared for that stair master. I kept telling myself that it wasn't going to be as bad as yesterday. Welp, ten minutes into the stair master there was a voice inside of me saying, "YOU LIED" lol. It seemed like today was harder than yesterday. I began to think to myself, "will I ever get use to this?" It was at that moment that all these other thoughts started coming in my mind. I heard these thoughts loud and clear. Thoughts like, "you know it doesn't take all that to get in shape", "you don't have to come every day", "if you keep getting up early and coming to the gym you are going to get sicker." On and on those thoughts kept coming.

"SHUT UP!" I literally yelled out loud. Thank God no one was around me at the time because I would've been embarrassed. At that moment I just knew that I had to silence the noise and that's the first thing that came to my mind to do. The funny thing is, it worked. I no longer was getting the negative distracting thoughts going through my head. I felt so good about my self that I bumped the level up one and finished up the last ten minutes of the stair master strong.

In the sauna I began to ask God to keep me focused on my goal and my destiny. God has a funny way of answering us at times. Right when I prayed that someone came into the sauna and immediately began to spark up conversation. At first, I was like, "man God I just want to sit here and relax", but God had other plans. He knew I needed what this man was about to give me.

The man was older, and he said, "good morning young man, I see this is your second day here." In my head I was like is this dude stalking me lol. I answered back, "Yes Sir, I come at night as well, but I need to begin to do more cardio so I'm coming in the morning to do that." "Is that so", he replied, "well if you really want to lose weight, if that's your goal, you should try intermediate fasting." He continues to say, "that is one of the quickest ways to lose weight." "Also throw some fasted cardio in there and you will be at your goal weight in no time." I thanked him for that information, and he ended up leaving out as he looked back at me and said, "I'll see you in the morning right young man." I responded, "yes Sir, bright and early."

Before entering the sauna, I prayed for God to help me stay focused and God turns around and sends someone at the right time to confirm what He had already told me to do. It's so encouraging when God does that. It reassures you that you are on the right track and that you will arrive at your destiny if you remain focused. I walked out the gym with my head lifted and a smile on my face. Things were moving in the right direction.

Though this was my second day in the gym, this was only my first day trying the intermediate fasting. I had decided to do my intermediate fasting times from 8pm-11:30am. For those of you who may not know what intermediate fasting is, it's basically abstaining from food for a specific amount of time. I decided to only eat between the hours of 11:30am-8pm.

Just as I had thoughts of the gym being a piece of cake at the beginning my mind said the same thing about the intermediate fasting. Oh boy how wrong was I about that as well, lol. Remember Mr. Distraction, well he popped his head up in a major way with the intermediate fasting.

As I'm leaving out the door to go to work, I was pumped up and ready to attack the day. I had just got encouraged at the gym and now it was time for me to go to work. My lunch was packed, and I had my healthy snacks ready to eat once 11:30am hit. I felt like I was on cloud nine, well that was until 9:30am. My stomach was in my back! I had never been that hungry in my entire life, at least that's how I felt.

I kept looking at the clock hoping 11:30am came quick. It felt like time was moving super slow. To make matters worse my co-workers so happened to bring in breakfast snacks and donuts. I don't know what it was but everywhere I went I couldn't get the donut smell out of my mind. Then Mr. Distraction whispers, "It's okay, you can eat one. It's not going to hurt you. I know you are hungry, just eat one. You can work it off tomorrow."

Again, I had to tell that voice to SHUT UP! This time I said it in my head and not out loud lol. I knew that it was nothing but a SCUD that was trying to take me off course. After I did that the voices stopped but I still could smell the donuts. I just began to drink water and I put some worship music on and that helped me get my mind off my hunger pains.

Finally, it was 11:30am and I could have my first healthy snack. You should've saw how fast I ate those peanuts and beef jerky. Even though they were regular peanuts and the original version of the beef jerky, to me it tasted like filet mignon. I was also excited because I had made it passed the first hurdle with the intermediate fasting.

The next few days went about the same as the first two. At times I almost gave up because the distractions were trying to come stronger and stronger. I just reminded myself that I must being doing something right because if I wasn't, I wouldn't be getting this much resistance. Remember this wise saying; you will never see a defensive football player trying to tackle somebody on the bench! If you are facing adversity, then that's an indication that you have the ball in your hand, and you must do all that you can do to score a touchdown.

Chapter 5

Do Not Despise Small Beginnings

A favorite scripture of mine is found in Zechariah 4:10. It says, "Do not despise these small beginnings….". This can be so easy to do as you are on a journey to a better you. Because we live in a "right now" society many people want to see results immediately. While for some things you may see immediate results, for most cases one must understand that it's going to be a process before you begin to see results.

It's funny to me how someone will watch a commercial on TV about exercising and see the machine or tool the person is using and immediately pull out their credit card and buy it. In there mind they have tricked themselves into believing that all they have to do is get the machine and they will automatically look like the model on the commercial with minimal effort. They fail to realize that the model on TV did way more than just twist back and forth on a machine.

What the consumer failed to realize is that once the machine arrives to their house, they are going to have to PUT IN THE WORK. That's why a lot of people have so many exercise machines and videos at their house collecting dust. They bought into the marketing but never got sold into the work it takes to get the desired results.

After a few weeks of the consistency I began to get in routine with things. The stair master had gotten easier to the point I had to bump it up a few levels. The intermediate fasting began to get easier and I really wasn't tempted as much as I was at the beginning stage. What really blessed me was after about a month in a half of consistency other people started to notice a change in my physical appearance.

I didn't really notice the change myself. Maybe because at the time in my mind I still saw myself as that 240lb person. Or maybe it was because I was so focused on the work and the journey that I really wasn't paying attention to the results. I will say this though, when people started noticing the difference it made me feel good. The compliments were very encouraging and motivating to me.

Up until this time I hadn't gotten on the scale since the first day I started my journey. I really didn't want to be discouraged by the scale if it didn't say what I wanted it to say. So, I stayed away from it in the beginning. All I knew in my head was the fact I was 240lbs and I had to do something about it. That mindset kept me focused. I think at that time if I would've hopped on the scale and saw that I had lost a certain amount of weight I probably would've had a cheat day that would've led to two, three, and four cheat days lol.

On the seventh week of my journey I remember coming home from my morning cardio session and I was getting ready for work. As I was getting dressed, I notice my pants fit bigger than normal. Even to the point where I had to make an extra hole in my belt for them to fit. This made me very curious to know what my weight was. I did not have a scale at home, so I had to wait until I got to work to check.

Even though a big part of me didn't want to know because of what I mentioned earlier, a part of me was curious because of the way my pants were fitting. When I got to work, I went straight to the room where the scale was and hopped on it. It seemed like it took forever for it to give me my weight. Suddenly 220lbs popped on the screen and I was in total shock! I stepped off the scale and then stepped back on. I had to make sure this wasn't an error of something. After stepping on it again 220lbs popped back up. I was extremely amazed. Twenty pounds lost in a matter of a little over a month. I walked out the room extremely happy with what I just saw.

Though twenty pounds is a lot, I still knew within myself that this was just a small step towards my goal. It's funny how after I saw my results there was a part of me that wanted to celebrate. I began to have thoughts like, "man I can have a cheat day now", "I'm going to get some ice cream tonight to celebrate". These thoughts only lasted for a moment before I came back to my right mind and realized I couldn't afford to celebrate like that.

Celebrating accomplishments, whether big or small, is okay to do. You just must make sure that the celebration doesn't actually be the very thing that cause you to go backwards.

Take for instance the word "cheat day". This is a word many people in the fitness field is very familiar with. This is when a person that has been on a rigorous diet and exercise plan is given a "cheat day" or cheat meal to enjoy. This meal usually consists of anything the individual wants to consume. As innocent as that may look on the surface, it's actually more dangerous than it appears if it's not approached with the right mindset.

When you have abstained from something for a long period of time your body begins to build resisters. This helps you no longer crave the thing that you once thought you couldn't live without. While this protective mechanism is good, most people fail to realize that your body also have memory cells. These memory cells are what hurt a person who have a "cheat day" but are not ready mentally for it. Yes, they accomplished a small step, and yes they should be celebrated, but not to the degree where it can set them back.

Once the memory cells get a taste of what it use to enjoy, it will begin to bring certain cravings back to your mind. That's why it takes a mass amount of discipline to celebrate in the form of a cheat day. I'm not saying it can't be done, but I am saying that if one chooses to have one then they must make sure their mindset is right and that they are disciplined enough to not give in to the memory cells.

"Wow, I lost twenty pounds", I began to say to myself. I was happy and proud of myself, but I knew I still had a long way to go. One thing I refused to do in the beginning of this journey was set a specific amount of weight I wanted to lose. I did that in the pass and once I would hit my goal, I would end up reverting back to the bad habits that caused the weight gain in the first place. Therefore, I was careful not to do that this time. I just took a quick moment to celebrate my small accomplishment and then I went right back to grind mode as I walked to my work station.

Never make the mistake to despise the small accomplishments you are having or will have. I don't care how small your progress is, you must understand that you are still PROGRESSING. I once heard a person say that a big shot is nothing but a small shot that KEPT SHOOTING. So, no matter what, keep shooting.

Chapter 6

Illumination

Have you ever heard the saying "There is light at the end of the tunnel?" I used to hear that a lot when I was growing up. Of coarse back then I didn't have a clue what my parents meant by that statement. All I know is that every time we came to a tunnel that saying would come back to my mind. It wasn't until I got older and began to go through different things in life that the saying started to make more since to me.

When I first started my journey, I couldn't see any change, but I still was feeling the pain of the process. It was kind of difficult for me because on one hand I was tired of my current situation, but on the other hand I really didn't want to go through what I knew I would have to go through to get the results I desired. I was in the dark part of the tunnel and it was very frustrating. I still didn't allow that to stop me from progressively moving forward. It was like something on the inside was telling me that it will all make sense very soon.

No matter what endeavor you decide to embark upon, you must understand that there will always be a "dark season" as you are on your journey. I'm not saying that it's going to be bad, but what I am saying is that you may experience a little uncertainty as you are moving forward on your journey. Know that it's normal to go through that. Just never lose focus on why you started the journey in the first place.

I remember being at the gym one morning and one of my workout buddies shared something with me. By this time, I had built a rapport with a few individuals there and we became gym buddies. We didn't work out together, but we did have that gym chemistry and we encouraged each other occasionally. This individual shared a principle that really stuck with me. He said, "Rome wasn't built in a day, but in the mind of the builder it was completed in a matter of moments."

Boom! There it was, the light had just turned on and I received illumination. Up unto that point I was wanting to see the results of the work I was putting in. When I didn't see those results, it seemed like it made it harder to push forward. Even though I didn't quit, in my mind I was very close to throwing in the towel. That key principle was the very thing that has help me grind as hard as I am. I began to see myself in the finished state I desired to be.

The mind is such a powerful force. It can enslave us or empower us. It can plunge us into the depths of misery or take us to the heights of ecstasy. The mind is truly a terrible thing to waste. I'm a strong believer in the saying, "if you can believe it then you can achieve it." When you have a made-up mind, there is nothing on this earth that can stop you from achieving whatever your intending to do.

The next month in a half seem to fly by for me. Maybe because I was no longer looking in the mirror daily checking for results. I no longer needed to do that because I had already saw myself there. The funny thing is, once I stop checking and just focused on the finished project many people started complimenting me on my outer change. It started to be a daily thing that people were asking me how much weight have I lost and what am I doing different. I began to share the different things I was doing, and many people began to ask me to help them get the same type of results.

I hadn't really paid that much attention to how much weight I was losing. My focus was more on my eating habits and the exercise regiments I was doing. On the fourth month I decided to get on the scale to see my progress so far. I was a little nervous because I didn't want to get on and get discouraged if it didn't say what I thought it should've. I figured if I lost 20 pounds in my first month in a half, I should at least be at about

205lbs by now from the 240lbs I was in the beginning. As I stepped on the scale my eyes bucked wide open! OMG! I was in total shock as the scale read 190lbs.

Wow, I lost fifty pounds in a matter of four months. I couldn't believe it at first. Even though I still had some ways to go I was extremely happy for where I was at. I finally began to see the light at the end of the tunnel. What's amazing to me about that saying is the fact that, even though there is light at the end of the tunnel you still must realize that after you get to the end of the tunnel the journey continues.

I'm not sure where you may be in your life at the time of you reading this book. For some, you may be at the beginning stage of the tunnel and it may look scary and challenging. For you I want to say, be encouraged, you got this. For others, you may be in the midst of the tunnel and you are experiencing much uncertainty. For you I also want to say, be encouraged, you got this.

No matter where in this process you may be, always remember that there is light at the end of it. You are going to come out and you are going to come out stronger than you were when you went in. Therefore, stay focused and continue to progressively move forward. Also make sure to remove yourself from any negative environment you may find yourself in. Negativity will drain your drive while simultaneously suck the very energy out of you that's so needed on your journey. You will be faced with challenges along the way, but rest assured, if you remain focused you will be okay.

As I stepped off the scale I began to think back on where I started from. I began to be thankful that in the tough times I didn't quit. I sat there for a moment at the end of my tunnel and game planned on how I was going to tackle the next phase of this journey. I knew I couldn't stay in celebration mode to long because I didn't want to revert back. I thanked God for blessing me and I asked him to help me continue to progressively move forward.

As I end this chapter, I want to share this quote with you, "Your tunnel will either define you or design you, but the choice is yours." I hope you choose wisely.

Chapter 7
The 30-Day Kick Start

I hope by now you have been encouraged and empowered to the point that you believe you too can accomplish anything in life. Even though this book is geared towards weight loss, there are many principles hidden in this book that can be applied to any area of life. I desire to see everyone that read this book win. Not only with your weight loss journey, but also in life.

I would like to now give you a 30-Day kick start program that will help you get started the right way. This is not the complete system, but it is a very helpful kick start that will help you tremendously. If followed correctly you will begin to see great results even after 30 days. May this bless you as much as it has blessed me and may this help you begin to enjoy the amazing life you were created to enjoy.

Plan In Action

Cation: Please consult your physician before jumping into any type of exercise or weight loss program.

This should be done with much focus and discipline. There should be sessions of prayer, meditation, and reading within these 30 days. There will be days that will be harder than others, but if you stick to it you will see phenomenal results. So, let's get started.

Action Plan

- Chose a time to wake up (Preferably early so you won't be distracted and can focus). Work your way up, start with getting up 15 minutes earlier than you normally do and then increase it as time goes on.

- Use this time to read, pray, and meditate.

- Drink a 8oz glass of water (room temperature) with 2 teaspoons of Apple Cider Vinegar. You can drink this while you are reading or before you read.

- Get some Mason jars (32 ounce) and some Yogi Green Tea Blueberry Slim Life. Fill jar with warm to hot water and use two tea bags. Drink on throughout your morning at home or at work.

- First meal should be between 11am-11:30am (Preferably a good snack packed with protein). I use P3 Portable Protein Pack (Chipotle Peanuts, Sunflower Kernels, Original Beef Jerky).

- Next meal should be around 12:30pm-1pm. This should be a nice clean lunch (Wraps are good, Salads are good, Fit Pop Popcorn is very good). Eat until you are full but not over full. Also make sure to drink water throughout the day (preferably half your body weight in ounces). Example: Someone that's 200lbs should drink 100 ounces of water per day.

- A nice snack should be eaten anywhere between 3pm-3:30pm. Make sure it's a healthy snack followed with water.

- You can eat another pre-dinner snack around 5pm-5:30pm. Again, make sure it's a healthy snack followed with water.

- 30 minutes before your dinner make sure to drink an 8-ounce glass of water with 2 tablespoons of Apple Cider Vinegar (very Important).

- Try to make sure that you are eating dinner around 7:30pm-8pm and no later than 8:30pm (this is very important).

Things To Stay Away from For Thirty Days

If you want to see massive results, then stay away from these foods for the whole duration. If you just desire moderate results, then you can have one semi-cheat day a week (semi meaning a "unhealthy" snack or two in conjunction to that specific cheat day, but still keep your times of eating.)

- All unhealthy snacks! Chips, chocolate, candy, pop, sugary items, coffee with sweetener (coffee plan is ok), bread (at a minimum wheat or whole grain), pastas for dinner, and alcohol (wine is ok as long as it is no more than two days out of the week. If you can abstain from it for the 30 days, it would be better).

Things To Do During These 30 Days

- EXERCISE IS A MUST!

- Try your very best to do some type of cardio in the morning. This is very important because it allows you to be rewarded double for doing something once. It's called Fasted Cardio which allows you to burn double calories for doing something once.

- Example: Say you run on the treadmill for 20 minutes and you burn 250 calories. If you do that same thing in the morning before eating anything it's called Fasted Cardio. The only difference is instead of you just burning 250 calories you have now burned 500 calories WITHOUT DOING ANYTHING EXTRA.

- You can add light weight training as well. Focus on more reps than on heavy weight. The focus it to continue to burn calories.

- Lastly make sure you get your rest. Rest is very important to getting results.

I hope this has help you and I pray that this journey takes you to new heights in your life. May you become the best you and may you inspire others to do the same as you embark upon this amazing journey. Hopefully by now you are connected to our private Facebook Group where you will be able to continue your journey alongside others who are on the same type of journey.

9 781654 305949